61495
—
32029

AF863177

Regeneration of Health

Nourishing Body Systems with Chinese Herbal Formulas

John Finnegan

Regeneration of Health

Nourishing Body Systems
with Chinese Herb Formulas

All rights reserved. No part of this book may be reproduced or utilized in any form or by any means, electronic or mechanical, including photocopying, recording or by any information storage and retrieval system, without permission in writing from the publisher.

© 1987 by John Finnegan
Third Printing April 1989
ISBN 0-927425-06-8

Published by

Elysian Arts
20 Sunnyside Ave.
Suite A161
Mill Valley, CA 94941

Table of Contents

Acknowledgements

Thanks go to my brother Todd for his good-hearted support, and to Jeanette Conley, Lynn Winfield, and Daphne Gray for their editorial input. Thanks also to Bruce Howard for his fine drawings and to Phil VanKirk for his invaluable design assistance and help in producing the books. My special appreciation goes to Kathy Cituk who did most of the editing and word processing in developing this book into its final form.

Introduction

Thousands of years ago the sages of China developed herbal formulas with special extraction and concentration methods that are among the most powerful substances known to regenerate and heal weak, deficient body systems.

Today's medical researchers are finding that elements like organic germanium[1], Coenzyme Q_{10}[2], hormonal precursors, and tissue nutrients are some of the remarkable substances in these formulas that give them seemingly magical properties.

However, there are certainly yet-to-be discovered factors in them, and no isolated individual substances have been found that can duplicate the powerful effects of these concentrated nutrients for rebuilding and balancing disturbed body functions.

Over a period of five thousand years Chinese doctors and sages researched, tested, and developed these formulas with unique extraction and concentration methods to perfect whole food herbal formulas which are unsurpassed in their potency and effectiveness.

These ancient sages had a very simple but surprisingly effective method for healing illness. They believed that most illness was caused by weakness of a particular glandular or organ system. They observed that the human body is composed of seven basic functioning systems: the immune, digestive, nervous, glandular, respiratory, muscular-skeletal, and circulatory-lymphatic systems. When illness manifested, rather than identifying and labeling tens of thousands of separate symptomatic disease entities and treating them as isolated events, they saw the illness as caused by weakness or imbalance of a total body system. They then fed the person the foods and nutrients that would strengthen and regenerate the malfunctioning system and the disorder cleared up automatically.

This particular viewpoint of understanding and healing illness by strengthening the gland or organ system which governs it is gaining more and more acceptance today. This is due in part to the repercussions of many modern therapies: both the public and medical profession are witnessing the damage from side effects that are often a consequence of symptomatic treatment of disease.

Ivan Illich, in *Medical Nemesis,* and many other authoritative researchers, have repeatedly demonstrated the ineffectiveness of symptomatic treatment. More and more physicians today are turning to wholistic methods of healing and some have taken a similar approach to the ancient sages—of treating disease by feeding and strengthening different glands and organ systems. This may be seen in the works of Henry Bieler, M.D. in *Food is Your Best Medicine,* William McGarvey, M.D. in *The Edgar Cayce Remedies* and Elliot Abravanel, M.D. in *Dr. Abravanel's Body Type Diet.*

The Shao Lin priests studied thousands of different plants and classified them into three basic categories:

1) Poisonous herbs.

2) Medicinal herbs to be used for temporary relief in emergency situations. (These have dangerous side effects and must be used carefully.)

3) Whole food herbs which supply nutrients that feed the glands and organs and help them to regenerate.

For instance, carrots and beets are whole food herbs that feed and help heal the liver; cabbage is a whole food herb that feeds and helps heal the digestive tract.

The Shao Lin monks discovered which food herbs had the greatest nutrients for regenerating a particular body system and combined them into formulas containing unsurpassed healing properties. It must be emphasized that these whole food herbal formulas are made from vegetables like carrots and cabbage and so are perfectly safe to use and work by nourishing the body itself.

The following is a compendium of some of the most potent of these ancient Chinese Formulas. These are exceptional because they are grown using organic methods in very fertile soils which provide the plants with an abundance of nutrients and the proper humus conditions for the roots to assimilate them. They are picked at a specific time during growth when the healing properties are at the greatest potency. They are then mixed according to the definitive formulas developed by the Shao Lin Priests through centuries of painstaking research and experimentation.

A primary factor in what makes these formulations so uniquely effective is the specialized extraction process developed for each herb. Many of the nutrients in herbs are bound up in the cellulose, in the complex protein molecules, and in other molecular combinations (fats, minerals) within the herbs. Ordinary boiling and other commonly used extraction methods only make available a small fraction of the herbs' healing elements. It is through the highly complex and specific extraction techniques developed by these priests that the nutrients are separated from their bindings with other substances and made highly assimilable, even by weak and malfunctioning digestive systems.

Special methods were then developed to concentrate the extracted substance to one-eighth its original size thereby making the formula many times more potent and effective.

All the ways in which these Chinese formulas help to regenerate the body will probably never be understood, but four principal functions are known:

1. They give concentrated nutrients that are readily assimilated by the glands and organs for use in tissue repair and regeneration.

2. They provide precursors for the glands and organs to use in their manufacture of key hormones and enzymes.

3. They provide basic elements (such as organic germanium) which release energy and oxygen at atomic and molecular levels.

4. They provide substances which feed the basic energy cycles, such as the Krebs cycle, in the body's metabolic processes to liberate energy, heat and oxygen.

---

1 K. Asai Ph.D., *Miracle Cure Organic Germanium*

2 E. Bliznakov M.D., *The Miracle Nutrient Coenzyme* Q_{10}

Formula 1

Tissue Cleansing & Energizing Formula

This is a very powerful deep tissue cleanser. It has been known to dissolve arthritic deposits, help break down plaque in hardened arteries, leach out heavy metals, break up cysts, help neutralize free radicals, and help remove parasites. It also has antifungal properties. It improves liver function, aids fat metabolism, increases energy, strengthens digestion, and improves nervous system function and mental clarity. This is a very pleasant tasting tea. Many people find that it is not only very beneficial to their health but enjoyable as well.

Begin by steeping one tea bag in a quart of boiled water for five minutes. Then start with one half to one cup per day after mealtime. Use only during the day at first. Once you have developed a feel for using this tea, experiment with concentration and amount.

Ingredients: Camelia leaf, Perrilla leaf extract, Mori bark extract, Alisma root extract, Imperate Root.
Caution: People with large amounts of stored drug or toxic deposits, or the severely ill should begin using the tea in very dilute amounts. It can cause strong cleansing reactions in some people.

Formula 2

Digestive Cleansing & Energizing Formula

This formula cleanses the digestive tract, kills yeast, improves digestion, and aids fat and cholesterol metabolism. It nourishes the nervous system and increases energy and stamina. It is especially good as a kidney, bladder and urinary tract cleanser.

People often experience slight nausea and intestinal upset initially as it kills yeast colonies and cleans toxic matter from the digestive tract. Begin by mixing 1 tsp. of powdered tea in 1 quart of water, and drink one to two cups a day. Increase the concentration of the tea and the amount you use as your system adjusts to it. (Many people use 1 to 3 quarts a day and find that it greatly enhances their sense of well being.) This tea has similar cleansing properties to Formula 1 and thus the same directions and cautions for use apply. If one experiences excessive discomfort, this can be mitigated by: using a more dilute amount, mixing it with dilute Formula 1, or taking it with food. (There is a trace amount of caffeine in Formulas 1 and 2 but not enough to cause harm to the body. [The amount is less than one-half of 1%.] Most of the caffeine is extracted in the processing.) The two teas can be mixed together to produce a beverage with much greater and more complete cleansing and metabolic effects.

Ingredients: Camellia extract, Lemon extract, Chrysanthemum flower extract, Jasmine extract, Lalang grass root extract.

Formula 3

Nourishing, Strengthening, and Regenerating Formula

Formula 3 is the most powerful herbal rebuilding formula known. It has a strong regenerating effect on the adrenals, reproductive glands, liver, pancreas, kidneys, and nervous system. It helps build up lean muscle tissue, improves fat metabolism and greatly increases stamina and energy. Athletes use it in large amounts to improve performance, and people convalescing from illness find it substantially aids their recovery.

It is the best formula I have seen for healing the mucous membrane lining of the digestive tract. One woman I know was scheduled for a colostomy after 15 years of deteriorating ulcerative colitis. She began using this formula, along with the other formulas, cancelled her operation, and recovered in a few weeks.

People with severe fatigue or blood sugar problems, and those recovering from addictions will find that it greatly stabilizes their metabolism and increases their energy when they use it several times a day. It is an excellent food for infants, as well, and will build up their health.

Formula 3 mixes up best in a blender. Maintenance usage is two tablespoons once or twice a day. For building strength or recovering from an illness, use two to three tablespoons three times daily. Mix it in the Tissue Cleansing & Energizing Formula 1, and take it with Metabolism Regulation Formula, Endocrine Glandular Formula, Korean Ginseng, and Women's Glandular Formula.

For weight management, mix it in Digestive Cleansing & Energizing Formula 2 and take a glass one-half hour before each meal, along with the Metabolism Regulation Formula.

It also makes great smoothies. Take this formula one to three times a day, and you will experience significant results. This formula is made entirely from organically grown herbs that are extracted and concentrated five to eight times.

Ingredients: Coix Fruit, Chinese Yam, Fox Nut, Lotus Seed, Lotus Root, Apple, Water Lily Bulb, and Imperate Root.

Formula 4

Respiratory System Formula

Helps rebuild and improve immune system function. It will strengthen the body's natural defenses and enable it to better overcome colds, viruses, and other forms of infectious illness.

The immune system and the glandular system are the body's main mechanisms for preventing and recovering from illness. Certain foods and food herbs provide nutrients which greatly improve immune system function. This formula, when taken with the Nourishing Formula, the Health Strengthening Formula, and the Endocrine Glandular Formula have shown remarkable success in regenerating and improving the body's overall health. Two to six capsules daily helps prevent or heal mild illnesses. Up to 16 capsules daily is recommended for severe or chronic conditions. Very severe cases can use 25 to 50 capsules a day for a short duration to aid recovery.

Ingredients: Mint, Silver Flower, Chuan-Xiong, Golden Bell Fruit, Chinese Catnip, Bell Flower Root, American Lovage Root, Angelica Root, Licorice, Bamboo Leaf, Burdock Seed, and Reed Seed.

Formula 5

Health Strengthening Formula

This formula nourishes and improves liver function and feeds the immune system, aiding increased production of T-cells. T-cells are immune system cells that fight infection and play a major role in regulation of allergic response to invading organisms. Using this formula to nourish and strengthen the liver and improve T-cell production often results in an improved capacity to fight infections, identify and break down growths and normalize allergic reactions. Many people with severe immune system disorders have experienced very effective help in recovering by using the Respiratory System and Health Strengthening Formulas in large amounts: the specific ailments include chronic mucocutaneous Candida Albicans infections of the digestive tract, throat, sinuses, vaginal areas and skin, and others with universal reactor syndrome, chronic respiratory disorders and immune dysfunction conditions. Recommended dosage is the same as for Formula 4.

Ingredients: Chinese white flower, Paris herb, Scutellaria herb, Dandelion, and Imperate root.

Formula 6

Endocrine Glandular Formula

This preparation feeds and improves functions of the endocrine glands, including the adrenals, thyroid, and reproductive glands. These glands produce hormones which are essential to life and regulate all the body's major functions and energy cycles. Among these are the blood sugar level, protein assimilation and muscle building, nervous system function, mental well-being, immune system function, detoxification of poisons, digestive processes, body stamina, body temperature and other essential body processes.

Many illnesses, from arthritis to a susceptibility to recurrent infectious diseases and many vague bodily disorders such as fatigue, overweight, poor digestion and poor nervous system strength, are caused by weak or underfunctioning glands. Strengthening and improving their function often clears up a whole host of disorders and dramatically improves overall body health and personal enjoyment of living. This has been well documented by many authoritative researchers including: Broda Barnes, M.D. in *Hypothyroidism: The Unsuspected Illness,* Stephen Langer, M.D., in *Solved: The Riddle of Illness,* J.W. Tintera, M.D. in *Hypoadrenocorticism,* Ray Peat, Ph.D. in *Nutrition for Women,* and others.

This Endocrine Formula, as well as the Women's Glandular Formula, the Korean Ginseng Extract Formula, the Tissue Cleansing and Energizing Formula 1, the Metabolism Regulation Formula, and the Nourishing Formula have all demonstrated safe, repeated success in feeding and improving function of the endocrine glands. Irregular menstruation, PMS and menopausal symptoms have been greatly helped when taken along with the Women's Glandular Formula. Recommended dosage is three to six capsules a day for mild to moderate conditions and up to 12 daily for severe conditions. Pregnant women should not take more than one capsule a day, as it might contribute to the baby's development as unusually large and cause difficult delivery.

Ingredients: Chinese Yam, Forty-Knot Root, Leek Seed, Poria (mushroom powder), Cornel Fruit, Paper Mulberry, Eucommia Bark, Mongoliavine Fruit, Morinda Root, Broom Rape, Senega Root, Fennel Seed and Lycium Fruit.

Formula 7

Digestive System Formula

Feeds and helps heal the digestive tract. Cases of poor assimilation, lack of enzymes, excess or insufficient hydrochloric acid, and intestinal irritability can be greatly improved with the use of this formula. This formula does not work by providing additional digestive enzymes, though many digestive remedies take that approach. Instead, this formula feeds and strengthens the stomach and the supporting digestive organs, so that their production of enzymes and acid secretions can be normalized and restored. Three to six capsules daily for mild to modesrate conditions, and up to 12 per day for severe or chronic conditions.

Ingredients: Ginseng Root, Atractylodis Root, Poria (mushroom powder), Licorice, Pinelliae Root, Orange Peel, Cinnamon Bark, Fennel Seed, Amomum Seed, and Mint.

Formula 9

Circulatory System Formula

Poor circulation is a factor in many illnesses. A decreased blood supply to the brain and nervous system will cause depression and poor memory. A diminished blood supply to body tissues and organs will cause a decreased amount of oxygen and nutrients, and a buildup of toxins which will create the conditions favorable for all types of disease to develop.

This formula increases vascular elasticity and helps heal circulatory disorders including varicose veins, hardening of the arteries, blood pressure malfunctions, excessive fat and cholesterol levels, and will also improve eyesight.Use three to six capsules daily for mild to moderate conditions and prevention of illness. Use up to 16 capsules per day for severe or chronic conditions.

Ingredients: Cassia Tora Seed, Gou Teng, Sophora Flower, Chrysanthemum Flower, Orange Peel, Pinelliae Root, Dwarf Lilly, Turf Root, Poria (mushroom powder), Ginger Root, and Ginseng Root.

Formula 9

Five Systems Formula

This ancient and comprehensive formula was designed to nourish and strengthen the five major systems of the body. It provides key nutrients to the Endocrine Glandular, Respiratory, Circulatory, Digestive, and Liver-Immune (Health Strengthening) systems. This formula increases the strength and proper functioning of the entire body.

Those who are ill take it several times a day to build up their health, while healthy people and athletes take it, along with the Nourishing and Cleansing Formulas to stay strong and fit.

Ingredients: Chinese White Flower, Scutellaria Herb, Dandelion Root, Gou Teng, Licorice Root, Tora Seed, Mint Herb, Paris Herb, Orange Peel, Coix Fruit, Fennel Seed, Cinnamon Bark, Poria (mushroom powder), Chinese Yam, Ginger Root, Barren Wort Herb, Hawthorn Berry, Chuan Xiong Root, Mongoliavine Fruit, Golden Bell Fruit, Sophora Flower, Fung Fong Root, Ginseng Root, Honey Suckle Flower (Silver Flower), Yuan-Hu Root, Ostrea Shell, Chrysanthemum Flower, Dipsace Root, Angelica Root, Alpina Ginger Root, Angelica Centis Root, Leek Seed, Balloon Flower Root, Bamboo Leaf, Dwarf Lilly Turf Root, Paper Mulberry, Senega Root, Imperate Root, Connel Fruit, Forty-Knot Root, Burdock Fruit, Cnidium Fruit, Reed Root, Rhubarb Root, Broom Rape Herb, Chinese Catnip, Asias Herb, Bai-Zhu Root, Boxthorn Fruit, Eucommia Bark and Morinda Root.

Formula 10

Women's Glandular Formula

This formula strengthens the endocrine glandular system and nourishes and improves the growth and healing processes. It specifically feeds the female hormonal system and often has a remarkable effect on improving PMS and menopausal symptoms. It increases energy and helps calm and stabilize the nervous system.

A pleasant side effect of strengthening the body's glandular systems is the improvement of skin tone, complexion, and beauty. People often say that their faces become ten to fifteen years younger looking within a few months of using this formula, along with the other formulas.

One mother's experience demonstrates the capacity of this formula to nourish overall bodily regeneration. Her sixteen month old child had been ill and failed to grow at all in the previous 6 months. The mother cut the tablet into little slivers, put them on his almond butter sandwiches, and in the next month he grew an inch.

Many people find this formula to be very strengthening and healing. For maintenance purposes use one tablet daily with meals, and for more therapeutic uses take 2 tablets daily.

Formula 10 contains extract of real pearl, which has traditionally been revered in the Orient as a source of special elements that rejuvenate the body's vital processes.

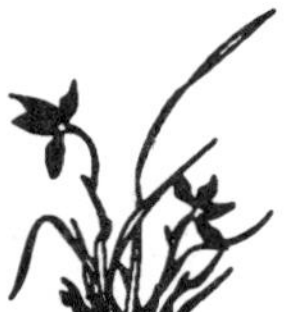

Ingredients: Honey, Korean Ginseng, Chrysanthemum Flower Extract, Royal Jelly Extract, Pearl, and other herbs as flavoring.

Metabolism Regulation Formula

A very powerful preparation with broad effects on many body functions. Excellent for weight management, it helps restore normal fat metabolism function. Many people report not only a loss of excess fat but a building up of lean muscle tissue as well. It picks up stamina and overall body energy, is a superlative cleanser of the digestive tract, and also improves the spleen-pancreas, liver, digestive, and glandular functions. This formula is also great for building up muscle tissue and strength in those who are underweight. Formula 11 consists of three separate formulations, to be taken together two to three times daily in a dosage of two to three capsules of each according to individual need.

Ingredients: Chinese yam, Taro powder, Plantago Asiatic, Tora Seed Powder, Camellia leaf extract, Imperate root extract, Caulis Hocquartial extract, Rhizoma Alismatis extract, Brigham tea extract, Senna seed extract, Rehmannia Glutinosa extract, Cortex Mori Radicus extract and other herbs as flavoring.

Formula 12

Healing Balm

Developed by the Shao Lin monks to aid recovery from injuries sustained during martial arts training. It was later found to be helpful for numerous other conditions, including insect bites, back pain, stiff neck, sore throat, heavy chest due to cold or flu, toothache, and sinus congestion. One nurse had a patient with a severe strep throat that was not responding to antibiotic treatment. She applied the balm to the sides of his neck, and within minutes there was tremendous improvement. For headaches apply to temples and back of neck. For sprains, bruises, minor arthritis and bursitis pains, rub into affected areas. Formula 12 also helps heal cuts, burns, sunburn, and minor infections. Many people get relief from motion sickness by putting a bit on the tip of the tongue and the back of the neck.

Ingredients: Menthol, camphor (2-5%), Cassia oil, plus other oils as fragrance.

Formulas 13, 14, & 15

Nervous System Formulas

Scientific research today is turning up evidence supporting what the Chinese sage doctors knew thousands of years ago. Recent studies on the health and functioning of the nervous system have discovered that certain key nutrients, neurotransmitters, prostaglandins, and hormones are essential to normal nervous system perception and function.

Stress, poor nutrition, poisons and genetic impairment can all contribute to creating a deficiency of these substances which will, in turn, cause serious malfunction of the nervous system.

The works of Dr. Fox in *DLPA*, Judy Graham in *Evening Primrose Oil*, Dr. Langer in *Solved: The Riddle of Illness*, and others have clearly shown the critical effect that these substances can have in clearing up depression, fatigue and phobias, and in alleviating the pain of arthritis and other diseases by strengthening nervous system function.

Today's pharmaceutical pain killers work by deadening the nervous system, and all have certain side effects. Proper use of nutrients and food herb formulas work by nourishing, normalizing and increasing the capacity of the nervous system to function well under stress.

While there is clearly a place for using individual substances in improving nervous system function, the most important thing is to provide complete nourishment of all essential nutrients through the use of whole foods and whole food extracts.

The importance of calcium in maintaining normal nervous system functioning is well known, but what is not so well known is the difference in absorption and utilization of commonly used supplemental calcium products as opposed to calcium taken from whole foods.

A recent study on human absorption showed that test subjects failed to absorb 93% to 100% of calcium from calcium carbonate and oyster shell.

This same principle of the significant difference in absorption and utilization of nutrients from foods and food concentrates, as opposed to isolated or synthesized nutrients, applies to most nutrients and is a major reason why foods and food extracts have such superior healing properties.

Since the endocrine glandular system (mainly the thyroid, adrenals, and reproductive glands) contributes at least 50% of the strength of the nervous system, the basic program should provide ample amounts of the Nourishing, Endocrine, and Women's Glandular Formulas along with the Cleansing teas #1 and #2.

General Nervous System Formula #13

This is the basic formula for strengthening nervous system function. Its use is indicated in conditions of general pain, burn out, and arthritis. It is used to aid mental concentration and perception. Dosage is 2 to 3 capsules once or twice daily, and more often during serious illness.

Ingredients: Cassia Tora Seed, Gou Teng, Ji Tsau Herb, Sophora Flower, Yeuan Wu Root, Orange Peel, Pinelliae Root.

Mental Clarity Formula #14

This formula is used with Formula 13 to enhance mental acuity. People who work with computers and bookkeeping have reported that by using 2 or 3 capsules of #14, along with 2 capsules of #13, they can work twice as long without mental fatigue. This formula is also good for headaches, neck and shoulder tension, insomnia, and mental difficulties. People recovering from addictions have reported it gives them great relief from mental clamor.

People with allergies have reported that using Formula 14, along with Formula 13, the Respiratory System, Health Strengthening, and Endocrine Glandular Formulas has cleared up their allergic conditions. Besides giving immediate relief, continued use over a period of time will help the body to heal the underlying disorder and aid permanent recovery. Dosage is 2 to 3 capsules once or twice daily, and more often during serious illness.

Ingredients: Mint, Silver Flower, Chuan-Xiong Root, Yeuan Wu Root, Angelica Root, Golden Bell Fruit, Ji Tsau Herb, White Willow Bark.

Joint & Injury Formula #15

This formula is used for pain from injury, trauma, and in muscle and joint deterioration. It is usually used with Formula 13 to give supportive nutrients. Research into the function of neurotransmitters has shown how critical it is to have adequate nervous system nutrients to help heal injury and clear up pain. Dosage is 2 to 3 capsules once or twice daily and more often during serious illness.

Ingredients: Siberian Ginseng, White Willow Bark, Mint, Silver Flower, Yeuan Wu Root, Chuan Xiong root, Angelica root, Golden Bell Fruit.

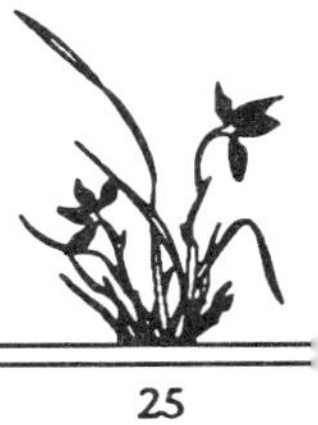

Formula 16

Throat Lozenges

The mouth, throat and sinuses can harbor the growth of many types of pathogenic bacterias, viruses, and yeasts. These can cause everything from sore throats and thrush, to tooth decay and sinusitis. The ancient Chinese herbalists knew what modern medical researchers are just discovering. Different plant oils have very powerful antibacterial, antiviral and antifungal capacities. These oils also strengthen the tissues themselves. Singers and public speakers say they can sing and speak twice as long when using these lozenges. Use as needed.

Ingredients: Gum Acacia, Sorbitol, Mint, Thyme, Eucalyptus, and other herbs for flavoring.

Formula 17

Sugar Craving Formula

A healthy, well-nourished organism is physically satisfied and has no unnatural cravings for sugar or other stimulating, addictive substances. Sugar cravings can be caused by low endorphin levels, low endocrine hormones, nutritional deficiencies (especially B vitamins and zinc), low blood sugar, lack of exercise, and the yeast overgrowth syndrome. Effectively dealing with sugar cravings requires correcting the root causes and often needs a complete nutritional, glandular rejuvenating, and antiyeast overgrowth program.

One traditional Chinese herbal formula that corrects

many of the nutritional and metabolic imbalances is the Sugar Craving Formula. This formula is very helpful, especially when used with a complete program.

Ingredients: Lycii Fruit, Wuxue Teng, Coix Fruit, Lotus Seed, Lotus Root, Water Lily Bulb, Imperate Root, Fox Nut.

Formula 18

Hair Tonic Formula

Growth, health, strength, thickness and beauty of hair is governed by many factors. One's genetic heritage, glandular strength and balance, liver function, and proper consumption of protein, B Vitamins, minerals, and essential fatty acids all play key roles.

Excessive hair loss or lack of luster can be caused by a weakness or imbalance of the endocrine glands and liver, as well as by nutritional deficiencies. Formulas that help nourish and strengthen the body's growth of hair are the Nourishing Formula, Tissue Cleansing Formula, Endocrine Glandular Formula, Women's Glandular Formula, and the Metabolism Regulation Formula. Foods that will also help hair growth are the Omega Nutrition Flax Seed Oil, eggs, Brewer's yeast, seaweed, and other good sources of minerals.

The Chinese also have developed a special combination of herbs that helps stimulate circulation in the scalp, nourish hair cell roots, and promote the growth and luxuriance of hair.

Ingredients: Water, Alcohol, Chinese Red Ginseng Extract, Astragalus Root Extract, Angelica Root Extract, Wild Ginger Extract, Ligusticum Root Extract, Chinese Red Flower Extract, Peach Nut Extract.

Beneficial Intestinal Flora

A complete colonization of the digestive tract with all the beneficial intestinal floras is an essential part of a healthy functioning human body. A normal adult has three types of beneficial intestinal floras: streptococcus faecium, acidophilus and bifidus. These bacteria are essential for human life.They help digest food, produce vitamins, and are a key factor in the body's control of pathogenic yeast, bacteria, viruses and parasites. They also provide other important but as yet unknown functions in the immune system.

Each of the three floras has distinct and critical functions, and an imbalance or deficiency in one can severely affect the functioning of the organism as a whole. For example, bifidus breaks down lactose, or milk sugar; a deficiency causes an inability to digest dairy products. In healthy infants, bifidus colonies make up 80 percent of their beneficial flora. [1]

Abundant colonization of the digestive tract with these three floras is one of the main homeostatic mechanisms the body has for controlling the growth and infection of pathogenic organisms. Proper colonization can be damaged by many things. The most common are stress, negative emotions, poor diet (lack of fiber and use of excessively refined and simple carbohydrates), and use of antibiotics, antiparasite medications, steroids, and birth control pills.

Proper implantation of all three floras is a foundation block of any holistic yeast recovery program. The quickest and most effective method is to ingest large amounts orally.

One company has pioneered the development of a coated acidophilus formula. One of the difficulties of building up a good intestinal colonization of floras is that the body's strong stomach acids can kill the floras before they reach the small intestine. This company has developed a method of coating the floras so they are protected from the stomach juices as they pass through the digestive tract. There are several companies making good quality acidophilus, bifidus, and streptoccocus faecium formulas.

Those who suffer severe yeast infection of the digestive tract need to take the floras continuously in order to gain control. This can take a few weeks or up to a couple of years, depending on the individual and the severity of infection.

An additional method is rectal implantation of the floras. Some people respond very well to this method. An important part of any vaginal infection treatment is vaginal implantation of acidophilus. Mix one-half to one teaspoon in warm water. Douche with a 20 percent solution of apple cider vinegar, then implant.

Regular consumption of good quality sauerkraut, pickles and yogurt is another important part of the flora replenishing program.

For those without dairy allergies, the best method of implanting large colonies of flora is to culture your own yogurt from one of the three floras and drink a half cup with one or two meals daily.

---

1. A personal anecdote illustrates the uniquely essential function of the individual flora. The six month old son of a friend suffered chronic problems from birth with digesting his mother's milk, with stomach pains, diarrhea, recurrent ear infections and sore throats. We started him on bifidus flora and all symptoms disappeared within the first day. He no longer spat up the milk, the diarrhea stopped, and he became a much happier baby.

Fiber

Our diets today contain less than one-third the amount of fiber contained in the diets of our grandparents, and in the diets of people in more rural areas of the world. The average western diet contains 10 to 20 grams of dietary fiber, while the diets of most rural societies contain 40 to 60 grams a day. According to the now classic paper that Dr. Denis Burkitt published in *The Lancet* in 1969, entitled "Related Diseases–Related Cause?," intestinal diseases which are prevalent throughout the civilized nations are almost unknown in rural Africa and many other societies.

According to Dr. Burkitt, most leading degenerative diseases are partially caused by an insufficient intake of dietary fiber. These diseases include coronary heart disease, diverticular disease, appendicitis, hermorrhoids, varicose veins, obesity, and diabetes. The second most common cause of death from cancer is cancer of the colon, which has been firmly linked to a low fiber diet. Even Candida overgrowth is associated with low fiber diets. While this information was reported in 1969, and nutritional healers have been saying these things since time immemorial, today we are seeing many articles about using oatbran to reduce cholesterol.

There are five known functions that fiber in the diet performs:

1) reduces intestinal toxicity and pathogenic bacterial and yeast overgrowth

2) improves bowel functioning and transit time

3) stabilizes blood sugar. It has been proven by many medical tests to help regulate both diabetes and hypoglycemia.

4) lowers cholesterol

5) protects against other chronic degenerative diseases, such as cancer of the colon, hemorrhoids, varicose veins, etc. Proper use of fiber has been firmly established to be the most effective therapy for clearing up hemorrhoids.

There are several ways to improve your dietary intake of good quality fiber: reduce consumption of overly refined foods; eat a salad every day with plenty of lettuce, grated carrot and other fibrous vegetables; use a liberal amount of whole grains and legumes in your diet; and, when needed, take some kind of high quality fiber supplement.

Additional Supportive Herbs

Goldenseal

This herb is superior for cleansing the liver and bloodstream. Goldenseal was considered to be the finest blood purifier and herbal antibiotic by such renowned authorities as Jethro Kloss, Dr. John Christopher, and several others.

Its use is especially indicated when one is healing excessive gut permeability caused by candidiasis. This breakdown of the intestinal mucosa is often a major causative factor of food and environmental allergies.

Goldenseal is an excellent herb to take during an infectious illness. It has been used effectively against respiratory infections, genitourinary infections, and against gastrointestinal diarrheas caused by E. Coli, Shigella Dysenteriae, Salmonella Paratyphi B., Giardia Lamblia, and Candida Albicans. Both human and culture studies have shown it to have significant amoebicidal activity against Entamoeba Histolytica. It has also been found to be active against Staph Sp., Strep Sp., Chlamydia Sp., and Trichomonas Vaginalis. Goldenseal's action against some of these pathogens is actually stronger than that of the antibiotics commonly used.

However, unlike prescription antibiotics, Goldenseal does not kill the beneficial digestive floras while it does kill candida and other pathogenic yeasts. This information was extracted from a summary of 29 medical studies describing Goldenseal's activity in the February 1988 issue of "Phyto-Pharmacia" included in the "Townsend Letter" June, July 1988.

People with infectious diseases, yeast disorders and ulcerated gastrointestinal tracts have found 3 to 6 capsules a day for one to three months to be of great aid in healing this condition. More may be taken during acute illness. Goldenseal should not be taken for more than 3 months nor used by pregnant women.

Korean White Ginseng

Ginseng is considered to be the king of tonic herbs. It feeds and strengthens the endocrine glands and overall metabolism. Athletes use Ginseng to increase their stamina, and people convalescing from illness use Ginseng to build up their health. It is used to strengthen the heart and normalize blood pressure. It also nourishes the blood, having a beneficial effect on anemia.

Its use is especially indicated for those with weak adrenal or reproductive glandular function, and those with hypoglycemia, fatigue, and nervous system weakness.

This herb has special catalyzing properties and will increase the effectiveness when used with other strengthening herbal formulas.

Three to six capsules a day is the recommended dosage.

Siberian Ginseng Root Bark

This herb nourishes the spleen-liver function and helps strengthen joint tissues, ligaments, and tendons. Traditionally, it has been used for lack of appetite, insomnia, forgetfulness, nervous disorders, low energy, and convalescent weakness. A review of studies in which Siberian Ginseng was given to over 2,000 healthy human subjects found that it increased their ability to withstand adverse physical conditions, increased mental alertness, and improved work production and athletic performance. In another review of clinical trials given to over 2,000 human subjects with a variety of illnesses, it was found to aid healing of both low and high blood pressure, improve adrenal and thyroid function, help prevent some forms of cancer, help heal many other illnesses and increase overall sense of well being. This information was reviewed in an extract from the Townsend Letter in the January 1989 *Phyto-Pharmica Review,* Volume 2,Number 1. Three to six capsules daily is the recommended dosage.

Chrysanthemum

This herb is used widely in Chinese herbal formulas. It has powerful antifungal, antibacterial and anti-inflammatory properties. It helps liver function, and traditionally the Chinese used it to correct blood pressure irregularities.

Stevia

Stevia has a long history of safe and therapeutic use both as an herbal sweetener, and as an antifungal, anti-inflammatory and antibiotic agent. It has been used for centuries by the natives in South America and for the last few decades in Japan and Europe, where it is much acclaimed by their medical profession as a dentifrice and a blood sugar stabilizer.

It is thirty times sweeter than sugar, yet has practically no sugar in it. It has been found to lower the blood sugar in diabetics and raise the blood sugar in hypoglycemics.

It is also remarkably efficacious when used topically for poison oak, athletes foot, rashes and infections.

Dong Quai

This is good for feeding the body's endocrine glands and improving the blood quality. This herb has long been treasured among both eastern and western herbalists. In the east, it is considered one of the best food herbs, and people cook it regularly in soups to increase their health and strength. It is favored by women to strengthen their glandular function, but should not be used during pregnancy. Recommended dosage is three to six capsules daily.

White Willow Bark

This herb helps to reduce pain and inflammation and improves the body's resistance to illness. Three to six capsules is the recommended dosage during acute illness.

Dandelion Root

One of the foremost herbs for cleansing the liver and blood. Indicated wherever there is a condition of liver damage, sluggishness or disorder. Also, where the blood is toxic or the joints ache. Three to six capsules daily.

Children & Chinese Formulas

Development and usage of these food herb formulas for 5000 years have given us products proven to be without toxic side effects. All of the herbal formulas are safe and beneficial for children to use. Many babies and young children have enjoyed improved health and well being through the use of these Chinese herbal preparations. Infants and children especially thrive on the Nourishing Formula.

The Respiratory System and Health Strengthening Formulas are especially effective for children. The dosage should be decreased by half for children aged two to ten; and one to two capsules per day is sufficient for infants.

Use of the two Cleansing and Energizing Formulas must be monitored carefully, as it would be hazardous to cleanse too rapidly or increase the energy of children too dramatically. Begin with small, diluted amounts for youngsters and increase gradually. The Nourishing Formula can be given full strength with good result.

Colds and Flus

A cold or flu usually goes through four phases: early infection, crisis, exhaustion, and recovery. During the early infection and crisis phases, eat mostly vegetable broths, herbs, and vitamin C. Healing should take place quickly with a minimum of suffering.

It is essential to eliminate all dairy and flour products during the early phases. After the crisis phase has passed and strength starts to return, begin to eat more solid food. Start with vegetable soups. Be cautious in consuming heavy proteins, starches and fats until feeling better.

Goldenseal is especially valuable to use for this condition. Use 12 to 16 capsules a day to speed recovery. Applying the Healing Balm to the neck and throat is also helpful. Use large amounts of the Respiratory System, Health Strengthening, and Endocrine Glandular Formulas, and drink lots of liquids including the Cleansing Formula #1 and the Nourishing Formula.

Sample Cold and Flu Protocol

Morning:

Cleansing Tea #1 with 2 tablespoons Nourishing Formula
1 teaspoon Acidophilus
3 to 4 capsules Goldenseal
2 to 3 capsules Respiratory, Health Strengthening, and Endocrine Glandular Formulas
1 Five Systems packet
(Optional for pain and allergies) 1 capsule each General Nervous System and Mental Clarity Formulas

Noon:
3 to 4 capsules Goldenseal
2 to 3 capsules Respiratory, Health Strengthening, and Endocrine Glandular Formulas
1 capsule each General Nervous System and Mental Clarity Formulas

Evening:
3 to 4 capsules Goldenseal
2 to 3 capsules Respiratory, Health Strengthening, and Endocrine Glandular Formulas
1 capsule each General Nervous System and Mental Clarity Formulas
1 Five Systems packet mixed in warm water or tea

Bedtime:
3 to 4 capsules Goldenseal
2 to 3 capsules Respiratory, Health Strengthening, and Endocrine Glandular Formulas
1 capsule each General Nervous System and Mental Clarity Formulas

Optional use as needed: Vitamin C, Zinc Lozenges, Cleansing Tea #1,Nourishing Formula, Healing Balm, Throat Lozenges.

Recovery From Addictions

People who have been addicts or alcoholics for a period of time usually have developed severe glandular weakness and nutritional deficiencies. It takes at least several months to regenerate their glands and build up their nutritional reserves. During this time, they need strong nutritional and metabolic support.

Every few hours, their bodies will experience extreme biochemical disorders, as their blood sugar drops, calcium, magnesium and zinc levels go out of whack, and their endocrine glands fail to produce adequate amounts of hormones. These biological disorders can create such pressures on their mental and emotional state that they feel severe depression and fatigue, and are compulsively driven to utilize sugar, caffeine, nicotine, alcohol and drugs for relief.

Replacement therapy is one of the main principles of this program. It is one thing for someone to try to stop drinking, taking drugs or using coffee and sugar; however, it is another thing for him to understand the metabolic disorder that makes him depressed, alienated, irritable or fatigued, and to have a formula he can use which helps heal the disorder.

It makes an enormous difference for a person in this condition who is trying to quit to have a replacement formula that will provide the nutrients his body is missing and give strong metabolic support to his weakened glands and blood sugar mechanisms.

One of the best features of this program is that it is simple and inexpensive enough for people to put together and follow with the help of their physician. It is important to work with a nutritionally oriented physician where possible, because the possibilities of low thyroid, yeast overgrowth and other disorders all need to be checked out thoroughly.

These Chinese herbal formulas have proven themselves again and again to provide the kind of support which helps people get off their addictive substances and into a wholesome balanced lifestyle.

Sample Protocol For Continued Nutritional Support In A Recovery Program

Before Breakfast:
Cup of Formulas #1 and #2.

Twenty Minutes Later:
Cup of Formulas #1 and #2 with 3 tbs. Nourishing Formula, 5 capsules of Endocrine Glandular Formula, 3 each Metabolism Regulation Formula, and 2 each Mental Clarity and General Nervous System Formulas. (Can also use 2 to 6 of Respiratory System, Health Strengthening, Circulatory System, Digestive System, Five System and Korean Ginseng Formulas if needed.)

With Breakfast:
One Women's Glandular Formula and 3 Digestive Formula.

Three Hours After Breakfast:
Tea Formulas #1 & #2.

Half Hour Later:
Tea Formulas #1 & #2 with 3 tbs. Nourishing Formula.

With Lunch:
3 Digestive Formula, 5 Endocrine Glandular Formula, 3 each of Metabolism Regulation Formula.

Three Hours After Lunch:
Tea Formulas #1 & #2.

With Dinner:
5 Endocrine Glandular Formula, 1-2 Five Systems packets, 3 each of Metabolism Regulation Formula.

Bedtime:
3 tbs. Nourishing Formula with 2-3 each of Mental Clarity and General Nervous System Formulas.

This is just a suggested outline. Each individual is different, and should determine the correct amounts that meet his or her needs through experimentation.

Managing Cholesterol

Hardening of the arteries is a newly developed disease of civilization. Coronary heart disease, which did not exist prior to 1900, now affects 66% of the U.S. population.[1] Remarkably, there are cultures, such as the Bedouins', who have lived for centuries on diets of mostly meat and dairy foods, and have never developed heart disease.

Today's conditions of hardening of the arteries are caused by lack of exercise, low thyroid function,[2] insufficient dietary fiber, deficiency of the Omega 3 and Omega 6 fatty acids, poor cooking methods, use of old food, chemicals in foods, free radical damage to blood vessel walls caused by poisons in water and food,[3] excessive consumption of saturated fats, and especially by the over-consumption of processed, devitalized fats contained in margarines, vegetable shortenings, and the highly-heated oxidized oils used in restaurant cooking.[4] People with high cholesterol should follow their doctors' recommendation and consider some of the previously mentioned factors as causes of their conditions.

The Cleansing Teas #1 and #2 are very effective in breaking down and clearing out plaque, especially when taken along with the Circulatory System Formula. The two teas also have a remarkable effect on improving the liver's breakdown of cholesterol. Including ample amounts of the Nourishing Formula, as well as the Metabolism Regulation Formula in the diet also contributes many of the nutrients the body needs for proper management of cholesterol production.

Sample Protocol For Managing Cholesterol

First Thing In The Morning:
Cleansing Tea #1 or Cleansing Teas #1 and #2

With Breakfast:
Cleansing Tea #1 or Cleansing Teas #1 and #2
2-3 tablespoons Nourishing Formula
3-6 capsules Circulatory Formula
1-2 Five Systems packets
3 capsules each Metabolism Regulation Formula
1 tablespoon flax seed oil

With Lunch:
Same as with breakfast, without the Nourishing Formula

With Dinner:
Same as with breakfast

In addition, as much of the Cleansing Teas #1 and #2 and Nourishing Formula as desired can be taken throughout the day.

Many people with hardening of the arteries, poor circulation, and high blood pressure have had rapid improvement in their conditions by using the above formulas and following the dietary suggestions, along with regular exercise.

---

1 *East/West Journal*, February 1988, "Butter vs. Oil" by Rudolph Ballentine, M.D.
2 *New Age Journal*, March/April 1988, "The X Factor" by Joseph D. Weissman, M.D.
3 Barnes, Broda, M.D. and Glaton, Lawrence, *Hypothyroidism: The Unsuspected Illness*, Harper & Row, NY, 1976.
4 Passwater, Richard, *Super Nutrition For Healthy Hearts*, New York, Jove, 1978.

Eating Disorders

Many people with eating disorders, such as anorexia and bulemia, suffer from severe nutritional deficiencies, especially zinc, essential fatty acids and B vitamins. They often have yeast overgrowth, as well. Also, they may have a low blood sugar and low metabolic rate, which causes them to crave something to pick up their energy.

Many medical researchers, including Dr. Carl Pfeiffer and Dr. Alex Schauss, have had excellent results by providing nutritional support to clear up people's disturbed eating behavior.

Several of the Chinese herbal formulas have shown themselves to be especially effective at clearing up the metabolic and nutritional basis of eating disorders. These are the Nourishing Formula, the two tea Formulas #1 and #2, the Metabolism Regulation, the Endocrine Glandular, the Digestive System, the Mental Clarity, the Female Glandular, and the Sugar Craving Formulas.

While there is no question that people often have emotional and social pressures which disturb their natural functioning, giving them the correct nutritional support often has amazing results, and can only be helpful in giving a person the physical strength necessary to deal with the stresses of life.

Weight Management

Chinese herbal formulas offer the only approach to weight management that works by normalizing fat metabolism, building up lean muscle tissue, and increasing stamina and energy, instead of by caloric deprivation. Most people are overweight, not because of what they eat, but through a malfunction in their bodies' biochemical processes which metabolise what they eat.

These herbal formulas work to nourish and normalize the functions of the glands and organs, so that the appetite will stabilize and the body will properly utilize the nourishment it is given.

When used correctly, these formulas will also build up muscle tissue and strength for those who are underweight, which can be a more serious and difficult condition to correct.

There are five factors involved in weight management: cleansing of poisons, normalizing the transit time of the digestive tract, increasing metabolic rate, normalizing fat metabolism and muscle tissue building, eating a good balanced diet, and getting proper exercise.

Studies have shown that when a person's nutritional deficiencies are corrected and the metabolism balanced, abnormal food cravings disappear, and the natural appetite for good food returns.

The best formulas for cleansing are the Formulas #1 and #2 combined into a tea.

The Formulas that normalize fat metabolism and build up strength and stamina are the two teas Formulas #1 and #2, Metabolism Regulation Formula, the Nourishing Formula, the Endocrine Formula, the Women's Endocrine Formula, and Korean Ginseng.

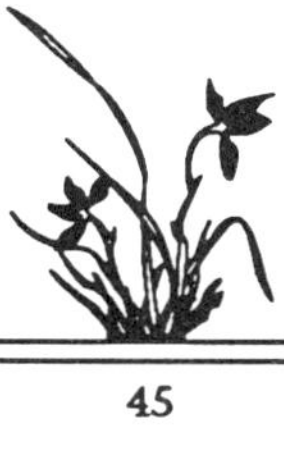

Following is a sample protocol for weight management which has helped many people.

Sample Protocol For Weight Management

First Thing In The Morning:
1-2 cups Tea Formulas #1 and #2.

Half Hour Before Breakfast:
3 Tbs. Nourishing Formula with 3 capsules each Metabolism Formula and 3-4 capsules Endocrine Formula.

With Breakfast:
3 capsules Digestive Formula and 1 tablet Women's Glandular Formula.

3 Hours Later:
1 or more cups Tea Formulas #1 and #2.

Half Hour Before Lunch:
1 cup Tea Formulas #1 and #2 with 3 Tbs. Nourishing Formula, 3 capsules Metabolism Formula, and 3-4 capsules Endocrine Formula.

With Lunch:
3 capsules Digestive Formula.

3 Hours Later:
1 or more cups Tea Formulas #1 and #2.

Half Hour Before Dinner:
1 cup of Tea Formulas #1 and #2, 3 Tbs. Nourishing Formula, 3 capsules Metabolism Formula, and 3-4 capsules Endocrine Formula.

With Dinner:
3 capsules Digestive Formula.

In addition, people can take as much tea throughout the day as they desire, and they can use the other formulas to help heal any other conditions they may have.

Initially, people will notice that they are losing inches but not weight, because their bodies will convert the fat to lean muscle tissue, which weighs twice as much as fat. However, as time goes on and they continue the program, they will find an increasing weight loss until they reach the correct weight for their size.

Arthritis

Most types of arthritis are very easy to heal. The main causes of arthritis are: calcium and magnesium deficienicies; deficiencies of the Omega 6 and Omega 3 fatty acids; toxins in joints caused by poor diet, poor liver and kidney function; weak thyroid, adrenal, and reproductive glands; malfunctioning immune system; lack of exercise; lack of adequate sunlight; both protein deficiency and excess protein; other nutritional deficienices such as zinc, manganese, boron, B vitamins, etc.; and insufficient stomach acid.

Rheumatoid arthritis is more difficult to help heal because of the malfunction of the immune system. The above causes apply, and the therapies listed below are quite helpful, even for this difficult disorder.

Many people get marked improvement from the Cleansing Tea #1. Also, the Nourishing Formula is very important for its liver, glandular, and immune system regenerating capabilities. Large amounts of the Endocrine Glandular Formula, and Health Strengthening Formula, are also indicated.

Sample Protocol For Arthritis

First Thing In The Morning:
Cleansing Tea #1

With Breakfast:

1 tablet Women's Glandular Formula

Cleansing Tea #1 with:

- 1 Five Systems packet
- 2 tablespoons Nourishing Formula
- 2 to 6 capsules Respiratory, Health Strengthening, and Endocrine Glandular Formulas

1 tablespoon cold pressed Omega Flax Seed Oil

With Lunch:

Cleansing Tea #1

With Dinner:

Cleansing Tea #1 with:

- 1 Five Systems packet
- 2 tablespoons Nourishing Formula
- 2 to 6 capsules Respiratory, Health Strengthening, and Endocrine Glandular Formulas

1 tablespoon Omega Flax Seed Oil

Diet should include lots of vegetables, both lightly cooked and raw, good quality protein, and plenty of fiber-rich foods. Cold processed flax seed oil can be poured directly onto food. Avoid citrus fruits and foods to which one is severely allergic.

Additional support of a good quality calcium and magnesium formula like Mezotrace is also recommended.

Application of Healing Balm to affected areas is often helpful.

Use Cleansing Tea #1 and Nourishing Formula as much as desired throughout the day.

Optional use of 2-6 capsules each of the General Nervous System and Joint & Injury Formulas, 6 capsules Siberian Ginseng Root, and 6-9 each of the Metabolism Regulation Formula daily.

Building Up Strength, Stamina and Muscle Tissue

There are two metabolic needs to be met in building up strength, stamina and muscle tissue. The first is to strengthen the endocrine glands, and the second is to provide all the necessary nutrients the body needs in highly concentrated, easily assimilable amounts.

Chinese herbal formulas provide the most effective nutrients for meeting both of these needs, and use no synthetic ingredients in their unique, organically grown whole food herbal extracts and concentrates.

Sample Protocol For Building Strength, Stamina and Muscle Tissue

First Thing In The Morning:
1 cup tea Formulas #1 and #2.

After Breakfast:
1 cup tea with 2-3 Tbs. Nourishing Formula, 4-6 capsules Endocrine Formula, 3 capsules Digestive Formula, 4 capsules Metabolism Formula, 3 capsules Circulatory Formula, 1 tablet Women's Glandular Formula, and 3 capsules Korean Ginseng Formula.

After Dinner:
1 cup tea with 2-3 Tbs. Nourishing Formula, 4-6 capsules Endocrine Formula, 3 capsules Digestive Formula, 4 capsules Metabolism Formula, 3 capsules Circulatory Formula, and 3 capsules Korean Ginseng Formula.

Throughout The Day:
Teas #1 and #2 alone and with 2-3 Tbs. Nourishing Formula can be used extensively. Some thin people do better using just tea Formula #1.

Smoothies

What a remarkable thing—something that tastes so delicious and yet is so good for you. Anyone who has boiled and drunk Chinese herbal concoctions is certain to have a special appreciation for the Nourishing Formula. Drinking a Nourishing Formula smoothie once or twice a day is a great way to increase strength, improve health and manage weight.

Put 12 ounces of Cleansing Tea #1, water, juice, or half yogurt and half liquid in a blender. Add 2-4 tablespoons of the Nourishing Formula, along with your favorite ingredients. Following are a few suggested additions to include in this delightful treat:

Some Additional Smoothie Ingredients

Almond Butter (1 teaspoon to 3 tablespoons)
Flax Seed Oil (1 teaspoon to 1 tablespoon)
Bee Pollen (1 teaspoon to 1 tablespoon)
Egg Yolk (one)
Amazake Rice Nectar
Yogurt
Bananas
Papayas
Cinnamon Powder
Acidophilus Powder
Korean Ginseng (3-6 capsules)
Endocrine Glandular Formula (3-6 capsules)

Almond Butter: An excellent source of protein, calcium, magnesium, and other minerals and vitamins.

Flax Seed Oil: Highest source of the vital Omega 3 and Omega 6 Fatty Acids which are deficient in most diets today. According to Udo Erasmus in *Fats And Oils*, these key nutrients are used by the body as a source of energy, to increase oxygenation, help prevent arteriosclerosis, improve immune system function, increase mental clarity and are essential to many other body processes. It is important to get only flax seed oil that has been extracted in a cold process method and stored in refrigeration in dark hard plastic containers that exclude oxygen and light to prevent rancidity. Normal dietary usage is 1 to 2 tablespoons daily. It tastes good and can be poured over vegetables, salads, grains, etc. See *Natural Foods and Good Cooking* for more information.

Bee Pollen: Has been called the most perfect food. It contains all the essential proteins, vitamins and minerals, as well as enzymes, and is easily digested. It lends a natural sweetness and substance when used in smoothies or in baking.

Egg Yolks: Raw or lightly cooked egg yolks are an excellent source of many key nutrients that strengthen and regenerate the endocrine glands, liver, nervous system, and immune system. The whites are excellent for building up muscle tissue and strength. When included in a balanced diet, they do not necessarily raise cholesterol levels; however, those with high cholesterol levels should be cautious in their use. The egg is one of the most nourishing foods and one of the best buys for the money. Many eastern sages recommend eating raw egg yolk every day to strengthen the entire system. Egg yolks have been recommended for those with nervous system and adrenal collapse. Add 1-2 egg yolks to soups or vegetables before serving. Be sure to wash eggs thoroughly before opening them, as Salmonella often collects on the shells.

Amazake: For hundreds of years, the Japanese have made a delicious, nourishing drink from whole grain rice called Amazake. It comes in plain, as well as a variety of delicious flavors, including almond. Nutritionally, the almond provides a good amount of complementary proteins, producing a great tasting drink with a substantial amount of complete protein. It also provides the key Omega 6 fatty acids and generous amounts of calcium, magnesium, phosphorus, potassium, riboflavin and other key nutrients. This naturally sweet beverage has no alcohol, preservatives or synthetic additives, no added sugars or salt, and has nearly all the nutritional benefits of brown rice. It can also be used as a milk substitute for those who are allergic to or have trouble digesting dairy products. Caution: Those with hypoglycemia or yeast overgrowth should avoid this product until their condition stabilizes, as it is high in natural sugars.

Yogurt: Yogurt contains beneficial bacteria, which help keep the digestive tract healthy. It is also an excellent source of easily digested protein and minerals. The Nutritional Almanac states the following: "Unsweetened yogurt contains the B-complex vitamins and has a higher percentage of vitamins A and D than does the milk it was made from. It is also high in protein. The beneficial bacteria in yogurt make it a natural antibiotic. Yogurt has been found to be beneficial in treating high cholesterol levels, arthritis, constipation, diarrhea, gallstones, halitosis, hepatitis, kidney disorders, and skin diseases."

Bananas: Have been shown to heal ulcers and strengthen the wall of the stomach. They are high in potassium, which benefits the muscular system, and pectin, which lowers cholesterol.

Papaya: Rich in vitamins A, C, and E, and is high in calcium phosphorus, and iron. It is rich in digestive properties, and is very soothing to the stomach. It is used in the treatment of stomach ulcers and fevers.

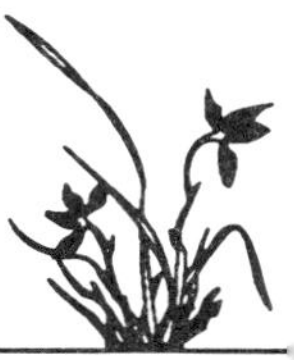

Cinnamon: Warms the system and is used to treat chronic diarrhea, cramps, heart and abdominal pains, coughing, wheezing and lower back pain.

Acidophilus Powder: A complete colonization of the digestive tract with all the beneficial intestinal floras is an essential part of a healthy functioning body. These bacteria help digest food, produce vitamins, and are key factors in controlling pathogenic yeast, bacteria, viruses, and parasites. They also provide other important, but as yet unknown, functions in the immune system. The digestive flora are damaged by diets high in sugars as well as by antibiotic and antiparasite medications.

Formulas For Specific Conditions

These formulas provide nourishment which strengthens the various glandular and/or organ systems, enabling the body to better heal itself. They do not heal or cure an illness. If you need medical care, please consult the doctor or health care practitioner of your choice.

Abscess:

Recommended Formulas: Cleansing Tea #1; 6-12 capsules each Goldenseal, Health Strengthening, Respiratory System, and Endocrine Glandular daily; 2-3 tablespoons Nourishing Formula two or three times daily; Acidophilus.

Diet and Additional Supplementation: Eliminate sugar and junk food from diet. Use 2 tablespoons flax seed oil, Vitamin C, and Vitamin E daily. Rub Healing Balm externally, and apply hot compresses. Take B Vitamins for 1-2 weeks.

Possible Associated Condition(s): Yeast overgrowth.

Acne:

Recommended Formulas: Cleansing Tea #1; Women's Glandular (1 tablet/day); 6-12 each Goldenseal, Health Strengthening, Respiratory System, and Endocrine Glandular per day; 2-3 tablespoons Nourishing Formula two or three times a day; Acidophilus.

Diet and Additional Supplementation: Eliminate sugar and junk food from diet. Use 2 tablespoons flax seed oil daily, and take Vitamins C and E and zinc picolinate. Take B Vitamins for 1-2 weeks. Apply facial masque with Stevia Extract.

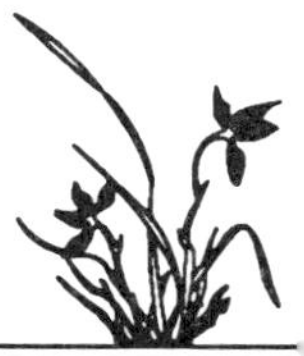

Possible Associated Condition(s): Yeast overgrowth, zinc deficiency, poor diet

Addiction:

See section in text on Addictions. Additional use of Vitamin C, flax seed oil, and Calcium-Magnesium supplementation. Use B Vitamins for 1-2 weeks.

Anemia:

Recommended Formulas: Cleansing Tea #1, 2-3 tablespoons Nourishing Formula twice daily, 3-6 packets Five Systems, Women's Glandular and Metabolism Regulation Formulas, Korean Ginseng.

Diet and Additional Supplementation: Eat organic liver 2-3 times a week, and eat greens every day. Include eggs, seaweed, and good quality protein in diet. Use flax seed oil, and Vitamin C.

Allergies (food, environmental, pollens, etc.):

Chronic allergies are caused by weak adrenal, thyroid and reproductive glands, poor liver function, yeast overgrowth syndrome, nutritional deficiencies, immune system imbalance, and poisoning of the system.

Recommended Formulas: Cleansing Teas #1 and #2 to tolerance; large amounts of Nourishing, Respiratory System, Health Strengthening, Endocrine Glandular, Five Systems, Metabolism Regulation, and Women's Glandular Formulas; also use Goldenseal (6-12 capsules daily), Acidophilus, Korean Ginseng, and General Nervous System and Mental Clarity Formulas.

Diet and Additional Supplementation: Eat wholesome, organically grown food. Use flax seed oil and Vitamin C. Drink plenty of fluids.

Other Recommendations: Reduce toxic load on the body by living and working in as unpolluted an environment as possible. Get exercise, and pursue a lifestyle that you enjoy. See *Yeast Disorders* and *Yeast, Parasites, and Viruses* by John Finnegan.

Anorexia:

See section on Eating Disorders. Also, use zinc picolinate, flax seed oil, and Acidophilus, and use ginger tea in cooking. Consider possibility of yeast overgrowth syndrome.

Arteriosclerosis:

See section on Managing Cholesterol.

Arthritis (osteo and rheumatoid):

See section on Arthritis.

Asthma:

Same program as Allergies and consider yeast disorder protocol.

Athlete's Foot:

Apply Stevia Extract locally. If condition is chronic, follow program for Candida Albicans.

Athletic Performance:

See section on Building Up Strength, Stamina, and Muscle Tissue.

Autoimmune Conditions:

See section on Allergies. Follow same program and consider yeast disorder protocol.

Balding:

See Hair Loss.

Bedwetting:

Recommended Formulas: General Nervous System, Mental Clarity, and Nourishing Formulas; Acidophilus.

Diet and Additional Supplementation: Avoid sugar products.

Possible Associated Condition(s): Yeast overgrowth.

Other Recommendations: Follow same protocol as for Candida Albicans.

Bladder Infection:

Follow same program as for Infection. If chronic or recurrent, consider probability of yeast disorder and follow same protocol.

Blood Pressure (High):

Follow same program as for Arteriosclerosis.

Blood Pressure (Low):

Recommended Formulas: Use ample amounts of Nourishing, Health Strengthening, Endocrine, and Metabolism Regulation Formulas. Use Cleansing Tea #1 and

Korean Ginseng.

Diet and Additional Supplementation: Eat lots of eggs, liver, fish, flax seed oil, raw cottage cheese, butter, good quality protein, and whole grains.

Possible Associated Condition(s): Low adrenal function.

Other Recommendations: Get plenty of exercise.

Boil:

Same program as for Abscess. Apply Healing Balm and Vitamin E externally. Use hot compresses.

Bowel Problems:

Recommended Formulas: Use Acidophilus, and ample amounts of Nourishing Formula.

Diet and Additional Supplementation: Eat fiber rich foods, yogurt, and flax seed oil.

Possible Associated Condition(s): Consider yeast disorder syndrome and follow same protocol.

Other Recommendations: Exercise.

Bulemia:

See section on Eating Disorders. Also, use zinc picolinate.

Bursitis:

Apply Healing Balm. See section on Arthritis and follow same program.

Cancer:

See Tumors.

Candida Albicans:

Recommended Formulas: Use large amounts of Cleansing Teas #1 and #2, Nourishing, Respiratory System, Health Strengthening, Endocrine Glandular, Five Systems, Metabolism Regulation, and Women's GlandularFormulas; Korean Ginseng.

Diet and Additional Supplementation: Avoid simple carbohydrates, and use lots of Acidophilus. Also zinc picolinate and flax seed oil are helpful.

Other Recommendations: See *Yeast Disorders* and *Yeast, Parasites, and Viruses* by John Finnegan.

Cholesterol:

See section in text on Managing Cholesterol.

Cirrhosis of the Liver:

Recommended Formulas: Use ample amounts of Cleansing Tea #1, Nourishing, Health Strengthening, Endocrine Glandular, Five Systems, Metabolism Regulation, and Women's Glandular Formulas. Use Acidophilus and Goldenseal.

Diet and Additional Supplementation: Organic liver, eggs, good quality protein, complex carbohydrates, greens every day, yogurt, and flax seed oil. Use zinc picolinate, and Vitamin C.

Other Recommendations: Eliminate use of caffeine, nicotine, sugar, junk foods, drugs, and alcohol.

Cold:

See section in text on Colds and Flus.

Colic (digestive tract):

Recommended Formulas: Nourishing Formula several times a day, Digestive System Formula. Five Systems packets several times a day. Cleansing Tea #1 for some people is helpful.

Diet and Additional Supplementation: Use Acidophilus several times a day, bifidus if for a nursing infant. Eat a good diet of whole fiber foods, high quality fats, complex carbohydrates, good protein and vegetables. Use yogurt, if tolerated, and flax seed oil.

Possible Associated Condition(s): Yeast overgrowth.

Colitis:

Same approach as Colic, especially indicative of yeast disorder syndrome.

Congestion:

Same program as for Allergies. Apply Healing Balm to sides of neck and throat.

Constipation:

Same approach as for Colic. Use lots of Cleansing Teas #1 and #2 and Metabolism Regulation Formula. Exercise and enjoy life.

Cystic Fibrosis:

Recommended Formulas: Use large amounts of Respiratory System, Health Strengthening, Endocrine Glandular,

and Nourishing Formulas; Acidophilus.
Diet and Additional Supplementation: Use flax seed oil.
Possible Associated Condition(s): Yeast disorder syndrome.

Depression:

Recommended Formulas: Use ample amounts of Nourishing, Endocrine Glandular, Women's Glandular, and Metabolism Regulation Formulas. Also Korean Ginseng, Cleansing Teas #1 and #2, and General Nervous System and Mental Clarity Formulas.
Diet and Additional Supplementation: Eat well and use flax seed oil.
Possible Associated Condition(s): Consider possibilities of low thyroid and adrenal function, poor liver function, yeast overgrowth syndrome, neurotransmitter deficiencies, nutritional deficiencies.
Other Recommendations: Pursue a lifestyle you enjoy. Find and develop a creative and meaningful form of work. Learn to love and accept yourself. Exercise.

Diarrhea:

Recommended Formulas: If temporary, use Goldenseal and Nourishing, Digestive System, and Five Systems Formulas. Sometimes Cleansing Tea #1 and #2 are helpful. Acidophilus.
Diet and Additional Supplementation: Use yogurt if tolerated.
Possible Associated Condition(s): If chronic, consider probability of yeast overgrowth syndrome and/or parasite infection. Use same approach as for Candida Albicans.
Other Recommendations: See *Yeast Disorders* and *Yeast, Parasites, and Viruses* by John Finnegan.

Diabetes:

Recommended Formulas: Cleansing Teas #1 and #2, Nourishing Formula, Five Systems packets, Metabolism Regulation Formula.
Diet and Additional Supplementation: Eat well, using good amounts of high quality complex carbohydrate,

and fiber rich foods. Use flax seed oil.

Other Recommendations: Exercise.

Diaper Rash:

Recommended Formulas: Nourishing Formula.

Diet and Additional Supplementation: Use bifidus floras in milk, baby formula, or Nourishing Formula twice a day.

Other Recommendations: Apply Stevia Extract externally.

Dysentery:

Recommended Formulas: Large amounts of Goldenseal (5 capsules three times a day) with Cleansing Teas #1 and #2; Acidophilus.

Diet and Additional Supplementation: Eat nothing but unsweetened yogurt, buttermilk, kefir and raw cottage cheese with herbs and lots of garlic for 3 days.

Possible Associated Condition(s): Consider yeast overgrowth syndrome and follow same protocol.

Other Recommendations: See *Yeast, Parasites, and Viruses* by John Finnegan.

Ear Infections:

Recommended Formulas: Healing Balm applied to neck and around ears. Use judiciously—too much can irritate skin. Do not use on infants or young children.

Other Recommendations: Follow program for Colds and Flus. Hot mustard foot baths, soak feet 1/2 hour 2 to 3 times daily in bucket of hot water with 1 teaspoon mustard powder.

Eczema:

Recommended Formulas: Nourishing, Respiratory System, Health Strengthening, Endocrine Glandular, Women's Glandular, Five Systems, and Metabolism Regulation Formulas; Acidophilus.

Diet and Additional Supplementation: Eat well, avoid sugar, refined foods, etc. Use zinc picolinate and flax seed oil.

Possible Associated Condition(s): Consider probability of yeast overgrowth syndrome and apply same protocol.

Emotional Instability:

Recommended Formulas: Nourishing, Endocrine Glandular, Women's Glandular, and Metabolism Regulation Formulas; Cleansing Tea #1, Five Systems packets, Korean Ginseng, General Nervous System and Mental Clarity Formulas.

Diet and Additional Supplementation: Eat well and use flax seed oil.

Emphysema:

See section on Colds and Flus. Follow same approach.

Endometriosis:

Recommended Formulas: Women's Glandular, Endocrine Glandular, Nourishing, Metabolism Regulation, and Five Systems Formulas, Cleansing Tea #1.

Diet and Additional Supplementation: Use flax seed oil.

Possible Associated Condition(s): Consider possibility of yeast overgrowth syndrome.

Environmental Illness:

See Allergies.

Epilepsy:

Recommended Formulas: General Nervous System, Mental Clarity, and Nourishing Formulas; Cleansing Tea #1; Five Systems packets.

Diet and Additional Supplementation: Eat well and use flax seed oil.

Epstein Barr Virus:

Ninety-seven percent of the population over 30 carry this virus in a latent form. It only becomes active when the body's natural resistance is broken down. Using therapies that strengthen health and improve metabolism is the only method that has been found to restore the body's capacity to control this illness. It has a symbiotic relationship with the yeast overgrowth syndrome, and most people with active Epstein Barr have the yeast disorder as well. Follow the same program as given for Candida Albicans.

Eyesight weakness:

Recommended Formulas: Cleansing Tea #1, Nourishing, Health Strengthening, Endocrine Glandular, Metabolism

Regulation, and Women's Glandular Formulas, Dandelion Root, Korean Ginseng, Circulatory System Formula.
Diet and Additional Supplementation: Eat well, and use flax seed oil.
Possible Associated Condition(s): Deteriorating eyesight is often caused by impaired liver function and nutritional deficiencies. Many have had their eyesight restored by strengthening their health.
Other Recommendations: Exercise.

Fever:

Unless really severe, it is usually best to let a fever run its course, as this is a vital part of the body's healing process. If severe, consult your physician or health practitioner.

Fertility (to increase):

Most of the time, infertility is caused by nutritional deficiencies of zinc, fatty acids, protein, B vitamins, etc., as well as by weakened adrenals, kidneys, liver, and thyroid gland.
Recommended Formulas: Ample use of the Nourishing Formula, Cleansing Tea #1, Endocrine Glandular, Health Strengthening, Five Systems, Korean Ginseng, and Women's Glandular Formulas will restore most conditions.
Diet and Additional Supplementation: Eat plenty of protein, especially eggs and fatty fish, greens, whole grains, nuts and seeds, flax seed oil, and nutritional yeast. Avoid drugs, sugar, alcohol, caffeine.
Other Recommendations: Exercise.

Gout:

Follow same program as for Arthritis. Eat only the best quality protein in moderate amounts and eat plenty of vegetables and fruits.

Hair Loss:

Recommended Formulas: Apply Hair Tonic Formula several times a day. Nourishing, Endocrine Glandular, Health Strengthening, Women's Glandular and Metabolism Regulation Formulas; Cleansing Tea #1.
Diet and Additional Supplementation: Eat a good diet

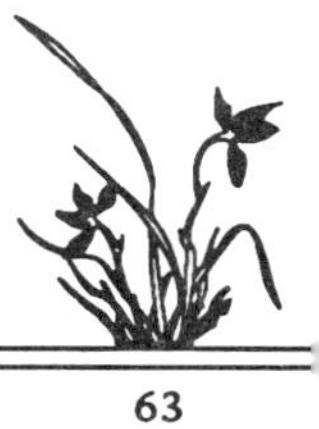

including lots of fish, eggs, brewer's yeast, seaweed, and flax seed oil. Avoid sugar, drugs, refined foods, and foods with chemical additives.

Other Recommendations: Use a good quality shampoo and conditioner.

Headache:

Recommended Formulas: For temporary relief, use General Nervous System, Mental Clarity, and Nourishing Formulas, with Cleansing Tea #1 and White Willow Bark. Use Five Systems packets, General Nervous System, Mental Clarity, and Nourishing Formulas, with Cleansing Tea #1 for long term rebuilding.

Diet and Additional Supplementation: Eat well.

Possible Associated Condition(s): Condition is usually caused by systemic weakness and toxicity. If chronic, look for underlying disorders such as low thyroid function, poor liver function, food allergies, poor dietary habits, yeast disorder syndrome.

Other Recommendations: Exercise.

Heartburn:

Recommended Formulas: For temporary relief, use Cleansing Formula #1, Nourishing, and Digestive System. For chronic condition, add Five Systems.

Diet and Additional Supplementation: Eat high fiber foods and use flax seed oil.

Other Recommendations: Exercise

Heavy Metal Poisoning:

Recommended Formulas: Cleansing Teas #1 and #2 are two of the best formulas for cleansing poisons from the body. Also use Nourishing Formula and Five Systems packets.

Diet and Additional Supplementation: Use large amounts of Vitamin C. Also use flax seed oil.

Other Recommendations: Exercise and saunas.

Hemorrhoids:

Recommended Formulas: Use Cleansing Tea #1 and #2, Nourishing, Five Systems, and Metabolism Regulation Formulas, Goldenseal, Acidophilus.

Diet and Additional Supplementation: Eliminate bad foods from diet and eat plenty of fiber-rich foods. Use Vitamin C and flax seed oil.

Possible Associated Condition(s): Liver trouble and circulatory system problems.

Other Recommendations: Exercise, and especially stretching exercises.

Hepatitis:

See Infections and Cirrhosis.

Herpes:

Use same program as for Candida Albicans.

High Blood Pressure:

See Blood Pressure.

Hives:

See Allergies.

Hypoglycemia:

Recommended Formulas: Use ample amounts of Cleansing Tea #1, Nourishing, Endocrine Glandular, Health Strengthening, and Metabolism Regulation Formulas, Korean Ginseng, Five Systems packets.

Diet and Additional Supplementation: Eat a good diet. Avoid coffee, drugs, alcohol, sugar and refined foods. Use flax seed oil.

Possible Associated Condition(s): Yeast disorder syndrome.

Impotency:

Most of the time, impotency is caused by nutritional deficiencies of zinc, fatty acids, protein, B vitamins, etc., as well as by weakened adrenals, kidneys, liver, and thyroid gland.

Recommended Formulas: Ample use of the Nourishing Formula, Cleansing Tea #1, Endocrine Glandular, Health Strengthening, Five Systems, Korean Ginseng, and Women's Glandular Formulas will restore most conditions.

Diet and Additional Supplementation: Eat plenty of protein, especially eggs and fatty fish, greens, whole grains, nuts and seeds, flax seed oil, and nutritional yeast. Avoid drugs, sugar, alcohol, caffeine.

Other Recommendations: Exercise.

Indigestion:

See Heartburn.

Insomnia:

Recommended Formulas: General Nervous System, Mental Clarity, and Nourishing.

Infection:

Recommended Formulas: Use large amounts of Cleansing Tea #1 and #2, Nourishing, Respiratory System, Health Strengthening, Endocrine Glandular, Five Systems, Metabolism Regulation, and Women's Glandular Formulas, and Korean Ginseng.

Diet and Additional Supplementation: Avoid simple carbohydrates, and use lots of Acidophilus. Also zinc picolinate and flax seed oil are helpful.

Other Recommendations: See *Yeast Disorders* and *Yeast, Parasites, and Viruses* by John Finnegan.

Influenza:

See section on Colds and Flus.

Jaundice:

Recommended Formulas: Use lots of Cleansing Tea #1, Nourishing Formula, Five Systems packets, Metabolism Regulation Formula, Goldenseal, Acidophilus.

Diet and Additional Supplementation: Eat plenty of vegetables, especially greens. Use Vitamin C and flax seed oil.

Possible Associated Condition(s): Condition is caused by liver and gall bladder blockage and malfunction.

Kidney Stones:

Recommended Formulas: Ample amounts of Cleansing Teas #1 and #2 will help break down and eliminate stones. Using Nourishing Formula and Five Systems packets on a regular basis, as well as eating a good diet, will work towards preventing their occurrence.

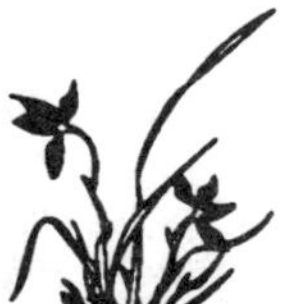

Ligaments (weak and/or torn):

Recommended Formulas: Cleansing Tea #1, Nourishing, Health Strengthening, Endocrine Glandular, Metabolism

Regulation, Siberian Ginseng, Korean Ginseng, and Five Systems Formulas. Use Joint and Injury and General Nervous System Formulas for pain in injured tissues.

Other Recommendations: Apply Healing Balm regularly.

Liver (damage and regeneration):

See Cirrhosis.

Lupus:

Use same program as for Autoimmune Conditions and Allergies. This information is not meant to be construed as a cure; however, nourishing and strengthening the body will greatly improve its ability to heal any condition.

Menstrual Cramps Or Other Difficulties:

Recommended Formulas: Cleansing Tea #1, Nourishing, Women's Glandular, Endocrine Glandular, Circulatory, Mental Clarity, and General Nervous System.

Diet and Additional Supplementation: Use Vitamin E and flax seed oil.

Menopause (hot flashes, dizziness, etc.):

Recommended Formulas: Cleansing Teas #1 and #2, Nourishing, Women's Glandular, Endocrine Glandular, Circulatory, and Mental Clarity Formulas.

Migraine Headaches:Recommended Formulas: Cleansing Teas #1 and #2, Nourishing, Circulatory , Mental Clarity, and General Nervous System Formulas, Acidophilus, Goldenseal.

Diet and Additional Supplementation: Good diet.

Mononucleosis:

Use same program as for Infections.

Multiple Sclerosis:

Recommended Formulas: Cleansing Tea #1, Nourishing, Endocrine Glandular, Health Strengthening, Metabolism Regulation, Five Systems, Mental Clarity, General Nervous System Formulas.

Diet and Additional Supplementation: Flax seed oil, evening primrose oil, gamma linolenic acid.

Muscle Weakness:

See section on Building Up Strength, Stamina, and Muscle Tissue.

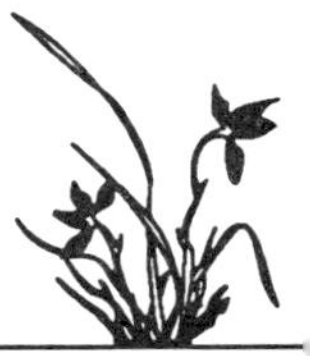

Muscle Aches:

Recommended Formulas: Cleansing Tea #1, Nourishing, Endocrine Glandular, Health Strengthening, Circulatory, Metabolism Regulation, Joint and Injury, and General Nervous System Formulas. Apply Healing Balm.

Diet and Additional Supplementation: Flax seed oil.

Narcolepsy:

Recommended Formulas: Cleansing Teas #1 and #2, Nourishing, Endocrine Glandular, and Metabolism Regulation Formulas.

Nervous Weakness:

Same program as for Neurosis.

Neurosis:

Recommended Formulas: Cleansing Tea #1, Nourishing, Endocrine Glandular, Circulatory, Women's Glandular, Korean Ginseng, Five Systems, Mental Clarity, General Nervous System Formulas.

Diet and Additional Supplementation: Eat a good diet. Use Flax seed oil.

Other Recommendations: Exercise. Find activities and work that you enjoy.

Ovaries (inflammation of):

Use same program as for Infection.

Phlebitis:

Recommended Formulas: Cleansing Teas #1 and #2, Nourishing, Circulatory, and Health Strengthening Formulas.

Other Recommendations: Rub Healing Balm on affected areas several times daily.

PMS:

See Menstrual Cramps.

Poison Oak and Poison Ivy:

Recommended Formulas: Stevia Extract is the best agent found for this condition. Nearly all cases clear up rapidly when it is applied to the inflammation. Also use Cleansing Tea #1, Nourishing, Health Strengthening, and Endocrine Glandular Formulas.

Psoriasis:
Use same program as for Infection.

Senility:
Recommended Formulas: Cleansing Teas #1 and #2, Nourishing, Five Systems, Metabolism Regulation, Women's Glandular, Korean Ginseng, and Mental Clarity Formulas.

Diet and Additional Supplementation: Flax seed oil.

Shingles:
Use same program as for Infection.

Sinus Trouble:
Use same program as for Infection.

Skin Tone:
Recommended Formulas: Cleansing Tea #1, Nourishing, Women's Glandular, Five Systems, and Metabolism Regulation Formulas, Acidophilus.

Diet and Additional Supplementation: Eat a good diet and use flax seed oil.

Other Recommendations: Exercise.

Sleep Difficulties:
Recommended Formulas: Nourishing, Mental Clarity, and General Nervous System Formulas.

Other Recommendations: Exercise.

Sore Throat:
Recommended Formulas: Cleansing Teas #1 and #2, Nourishing, Respiratory, Health Strengthening, and Endocrine Glandular Formulas, Goldenseal, Throat Lozenges.

Other Recommendations: Rub Healing Balm on throat.

Stomach Discomfort:
Recommended Formulas: Nourishing, Cleansing Tea #1, and Digestive System Formulas, Acidophilus.

Stress:
Recommended Formulas: Cleansing Teas #1 and #2, Nourishing, Endocrine Glandular, Korean Ginseng, Metabolism Regulation, Five Systems, Mental Clarity, and General Nervous System Formulas.

Diet and Additional Supplementation: Use flax seed oil.

Stroke (recovery):

See section in text on Managing Cholesterol.

Toothache:

Recommended Formulas: Mental Clarity, General Nervous System, Joint and Injury, White Willow Bark, and Nourishing Formulas, Cleansing Tea #1.

Thrush:

Follow program for Candida Albicans. Gargle with 6 capsules of Goldenseal in 4 ounces of warm water. Also gargle with hydrogen peroxide (being careful not to swallow it). Eat lots of garlic.

Tumors:

Recommended Formulas: Cleansing Teas #1 and #2; 2-3 tablespoons Nourishing Formulas two or three times a day; large amounts (12-20 and up per day) Health Strengthening and Respiratory System Formulas; Five Systems packets, Acidophilus, Goldenseal.

Diet and Additional Supplementation: Good dietary practices. Eat carotene-rich foods, and drink carrot juice. Use large amounts of pancreatic digestive enzymes. Also use flax seed oil and Vitamins C, E, and beta carotene.

Vaginal Yeast Infections:

Douche with 3 teaspoons of Cleansing Tea #2 in 16 ounces of warm water. If chronic, follow program for Candida Albicans.

Ulcers:

Recommended Formulas: 3 tablespoons Nourishing Formula in 8 ounces warm water three times a day, with 3-4 capsules Digestive System Formula emptied into it. Five Systems packets, Goldenseal, Acidophilus, and Mental Clarity and General Nervous System Formulas.

Diet and Additional Supplementation: Eat a good diet with lots of carrots and potatoes. Also use flax seed oil.

Other Recommendations: Exercise.

Varicose Veins:

Recommended Formulas: Cleansing Teas #1 and #2, Nourishing, Circulatory System, and Five Systems Formulas.

Diet and Additional Supplementation: Use Vitamins C and E.

Other Recommendations: Apply Healing Balm daily.

Viral Infections:

See Infections.

Weight Control:

See section on Weight Management.

Wrinkles:

Recommended Formulas: Cleansing Teas #1 and #2, Nourishing, Women's Glandular, Endocrine Glandular, Five Systems, and Metabolism Regulation Formulas.

Diet and Additional Supplementation: Use flax seed oil.

Yeast Disorder or Yeast Overgrowth:

See Candida Albicans.

An Understanding of Healing

The most important factor in a person's well being is how that person approaches life and how he sees himself, how he feels about himself. No therapy, herbs, medicine, or nutritional program will work permanently, unless a person is living consciously.

People are guided to those things in this creation which will help them when they ask for guidance. When people are trying to understand and live in harmony with how this creation was made, they are open to receive the support, grace, and care that is given to this life. That vision and clarity come from a true heart.

The first factor that is really important is a person's sense of self-worth. That is a tremendous factor in illness. People don't really see how beautiful they are. The beauty I'm talking about is the beauty of the life that is within. The life that is given to each person is so precious, so priceless.

Because you are the carrier of that life, you have worth, you deserve the care and quality of life, so that you can experience the beauty that is inside you. You can experience the fulfillment and the purpose of life. And you also can have the appreciation for all that is in this creation that is made for you to enjoy.

So often people accept jobs, relationships, and even the quality of food that they eat, just because they have been taught by their parents, schools, and associates to swallow it. It takes real work to develop a sense of self worth and a creative job situation.

Getting free is really important. It is essential to feel that you're worth the care that is going to get you well, that you are precious and that you deserve a pace that is healthy for you. So many people put themselves in situations again and again where they take on so much responsibility and try to live up to so many expectations, that they continue to burn themselves out.

Then they want to take some medicines or herbs to heal them. This approach will never work unless they heal the core issues which cause them to repeatedly overextend themselves, and to get involved in destructive relationships.

People deserve to feel good about themselves, to have time for themselves, and to have the basics in life, good food, and a comfortable home. We have to work for it, but we deserve it too.

People often sell themselves short. Some people are reacting to the greed, exploitation, and oppression they experience. They don't want to become greedy or exploitative, so they go to the other extreme and deny themselves.

The next factors are gratitude, commitment and responsibility. To get well when you are sick takes commitment, responsibility, and a real feeling of gratefulness for help when it is given. It is up to the individual. There's help, but it's your job. It's your work. When I say responsibility, I'm talking about the responsibility to yourself and to the power that gives us life. So much of the time we're taught there's a responsibility to our government, to society, and to our family and our friends. By the time we meet all our external responsibilities, there is nothing left for us.

There is a responsibility to society. I have a responsibility in driving a car to stop at stop signs, and not endanger other people's lives. I have a responsibility to respect other people's property and other people's lives. Those things are really important, but at least as important is my responsibility to myself and to the power that gives me life. It is not right to sacrifice, to compromise our responsibility to ourselves and to our life for everything else. There has to be a balance between our own self-interest and the laws of creation and society.

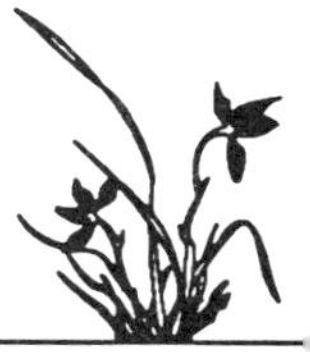

I've known people who were sent home to die with only a few days to live. Now they are completely fit and healthy. They're like athletes. I also know people who after 10 or 15 years have not been able to get over the simplest kind of illness.

The difference in those two people, is that one of them really started to take responsibility for his life. One of them really made a commitment and stuck with it. The other one fooled around, not really looking at the reality.

The third factor is knowledge. Say you're sick and you want to get well. You've taken responsibility, you realize it's up to you to find out what is really going on and to take the proper steps to get well. The next thing is to find out what to do, what works and what doesn't. That's what I mean by knowledge. You need to know what foods are good for you, what kind of lifestyle is good for you, what kind of job is good for you, what kind of friends are good for you, what kind of vitamins are good for you, which doctors can help you and which can't, and so on. This is the kind of practical knowledge that takes real study.

Finally, the fourth factor is wisdom. For most of us, wisdom is hard-earned and comes from mistakes. Sometimes we're smart enough to learn by listening. Most of the time we learn by making mistakes, often the same mistakes over and over again. We need to gather a sense of our entire condition. A simple example showing the difference between knowledge and wisdom is this: knowledge is the information that a drug is bad for you; wisdom is not using it.

Within the context of all these factors, these herbs are a gift in this creation. Somewhere it is written that, "...next to every poisonous plant is the plant that will heal that poison." If you find a stinging nettle in nature, next to it you will usually find dock, which when rubbed on the skin will cure the sting of the nettle.

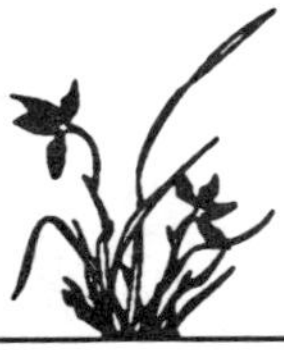

In the wisdom of this creation, the creator knew that we were going to make mistakes, and so also created things to help us when we made our mistakes. These herbs are a gift, and they are wonderful.

Bibliography

Abravanel, Elliot, M.D. .... Dr. Abravanel's Body Type Diet
New York: Bantam Books, 1986

Asai, K., Ph.D. .... Miracle Cure Organic Germanium
Tokyo: Japan Publications, 1980

Barnes, Broda, M.D. .... Hypothyroidism: The Unsuspected Illness
New York: Harper and Row, 1976

Bieler, Henry, M.D. .... Food Is Your Best Medicine
New York: Random House/Vintage Books, 1973

Bland, Jeffrey, Ph.D. .... Intestinal Toxicity and Inner Cleansing
New Canaan, CT: Keats Publishing, 1987

Bliznakov, E., M.D. .... The Miracle Nutrient Coenzyme Q10
New York: Bantam Books, 1987

Cituk, Kathy and Finnegan, John .... Natural Foods and Good Cooking
Mill Valley, Ca: Elysian Arts, 1989

Erasmus, Udo .... Fats And Oils
Vancouver, B.C.: Alive Books, 1986

Finnegan, John .... Addictions: A Nutritional Approach To Recovery
Mill Valley, Ca: Elysian Arts, 1989

Finnegan, John .... Amazake Rice Nectar
Mill Valley, Ca: Elysian Arts, 1989

Finnegan, John .... Yeast Disorders
Mill Valley, Ca: Elysian Arts, 1987

Finnegan, John .... Yeast, Parasites, and Viruses
Mill Valley, Ca: Elysian Arts, 1989

Finnegan, John and Gray, Daphne .... Recovery From Addiction
Mill Valley, Ca: Elysian Arts, 1989

Fox, Arnold, M.D. .... DLPA
New York: Pocket Books 1985

Graham, Judy .... Evening Primrose Oil
New York: Thorsons, 1984

Graham, Judy and Odent, Michel, Dr. .... The Z Factor
Vermont: Thorsons, 1986

Hsu, Hong-Yen .... Oriental Materia Medica
Long Beach, Ca: Oriental Healing Arts, 1986

Illich, Ivan .... Medical Nemesis
New York: Bantam Books, 1983

Keys, John .... Chinese Herbs
Rutland, Vt: Charles Tuttle, 1976

Kowalski, Robert E. .... The 8-Week Cholesterol Cure
New York: Harper & Row, 1987

Langer, Stephen, M.D. .... Solved: The Riddle of Illness
Connecticut: Keats Publishing

Lu, Henry ... Chinese System Of Food Cures
New York: Sterling Publishing, 1986

McGarvey, William, M.D. ... The Edgar Cayce Remedies
New York: Bantam Books, 1983

Murray, Michael, N.D. ... Phyto-Pharmacia, Vol. #2, 1988
Townsend Letter, June-July 1988

Peat, Ray ... Nutrition For Women
Oregon: Blake College Press, 1983

Pfeiffer, Carl, M.D. ... Zinc and Other Micronutrients
Connecticut: Keats Publishing

Prescott, Robert ... Chinese Keys To Regeneration
Draper, Ut: JBE Press, 1984

Prevention Magazine ... New Encyclopedia Of Common Diseases
Emmaus, Pa: Rodale Press, 1984

Reid, Daniel ... Chinese Herbal Medicine
Boston: Shambala, 1987

Rudin, Donald O., M.D. and Clara Felix ... The Omega-3 Phenomenon
New York: Rawson, 1987

Schauss, Alex, M.D. ... Crime, Diet & Delinquency
Biosocial Publications

Stoff, Jesse A., M.D. and Pellegrino, Charles, Ph.D. ... Chronic Fatigue Syndrome
New York: Random House, 1988

Tierra, Michael, N.D. ... The Way of Herbs
New York: Pocket Books 1983

Tierra, Michael, N.D. ... Planetary Herbology
New Mexico: Lotus Press, 1988

Tintera, J.W., M.D. ... Hypoadrenocorticism
New York: Hypoglycemia Foundation, 1968

Tsung, Pi-Kwang ... Immunology and Chinese Herbal Medicine
Long Beach, Ca: Oriental Healing Arts, 1986

Disclaimer:

This booklet has been written and published solely for informational and educational purposes, to provide insight into the value and possible benefits of certain traditional Chinese herbs and herbal formulas.

Please be advised that it is not the intention of this guide to provide medical advice or to substitute for the role of a physican in treating illness. The author and publisher provide this information with the understanding that you act on it at your own risk.

About The Author

John Finnegan, nutritional and environmental consultant, has spent twenty years studying and working in the holistic health field. With a college background in the life sciences, he went on to study and work with many of this century's leading medical pioneers. He studied and worked with Dr. John Christopher, Dr. Michael Barnett, and in several holistic medical centers.

John Finnegan is the author of five books, including *Recovery From Addiction,* and *Yeast, Parasites and Viruses.* He lectures and conducts seminars, and gave presentations at both the 1987 and 1988 San Francisco Whole Life Expos.

Elysian Arts presents . . .

Yeast Disorders
An Understanding And Nutritional Therapy
by John Finnegan

This 112-page book shows how traditional Chinese Herbal Formulas are having an amazing regenerative effect on the widespread epidemic of yeast-based and immune system disorders.
ISBN 0-927425-00-9
Second Printing

Prices

1 to 9 copies..........$8.00
10 to 49 copies......$7.50
50 to 99 copies......$7.00
Over 100 copies.....$5.00

Please send ________ copies

@ $________ = $_________

Natural Foods and Good Cooking
by Kathy Cituk with John Finnegan

Aimed at utilizing the maximum nutritional and healing properties of natural foods, this 128-page book meets a real need for information about food and cooking that is both simple and based on common sense as well as scientific fact. Besides a wealth of easy to prepare, delicious recipes, it features special sections on using oils and butter, salt, herbs, and spices, and other foods that will provide you with practical guidance on how to eat well
ISBN 0-927425-01-7

Prices

1 to 9 copies..........$8.00
10 to 49 copies......$7.50
50 to 99 copies......$7.00
Over 100 copies....$5.00

Please send ________ copies

@ $________ = $_________

Addictions:
A Nutritional Approach To Recovery
by John Finnegan

The purpose of this 160-page book is to provide an overview of the factors involved in recovery from addictions. It provides the most complete, up-to-date information on the metabolic basis of addictions. It also presents some of the most effective nutritional, herbal, and medical therapies, which are gaining renown for their ability to correct these biochemical disorders.
ISBN 0-927425-05-X

Prices

1 to 9 copies..........$9.00
10 to 49 copies......$8.00
50 to 99 copies......$7.00
Over 100 copies.....$5.50

Please send ________ copies

@ $________ = $_________

Yeast, Parasites, and Viruses

An Understanding With Nutritional Therapies
by John Finnegan

Newly revised and expanded, this comprehensive book includes major sections on Liver Function, Hormonal Support, Parasites, Viruses, Yeast Disorders, and much more.
ISBN 0-927425-03-3

Prices

1 to 9 copies..........$9.00
10 to 49 copies......$8.00
50 to 99 copies......$7.00
Over 100 copies....$5.50

Please send ________ copies

@ $________ = $_________

Regeneration Of Health

Nourishing Body Systems With Chinese Food Herb Formulas
by John Finnegan

This 80-page book contains in-depth information on ancient Chinese herbal formulas, Managing Cholesterol, Recovery From Addictions, Fiber, Weight Management, and an entirely new section on Formulas And Other Therapies For Over 100 Common Illnesses.
ISBN 0-927425-06-8
Third Printing

Prices

1 to 9 copies..........$5.00
10 to 49 copies......$4.25
50 to 99 copies......$3.50
Over 100 copies....$3.00

Please send ________ copies

@ $________ = $_________

Shipping Costs*

1 to 9 books..................$5.00
10 to 49 books.............$7.00
50 to 99 books............$12.00
Over 100 books..........$20.00

*Please note: Shipping outside of U.S., including Hawaii, Alaska, and Canada is double.

Book Total = $____________

6% Sales Tax = $____________
(California Residents Only)

***Shipping = $____________**

Total = $ ___________

Name ______________________________

Address ______________________________

City ______________________________

State ______________ **Zip** ______________

Please make checks payable
(in U.S. funds only) to:
Elysian Arts
20 Sunnyside Ave.
Suite A161
Mill Valley, CA 94941